How to Boost Your Immune System

An Essential Guide to Improve Your Immune System for Greater Health and Wellness

by Wena Armstrong

Table of Contents

Introduction

Your immune system acts as your body's defense mechanism against foreign bodies and invading microorganisms. Hence, it's vital to know exactly how you can promote its proper function. Your immune system is composed of several organs and processes that all work together in forming your immune response. This immune response is how your body is able to heal and cure itself, without having to take any medication. It naturally facilitates the healing of wounds, it helps your cells to eliminate harmful substances, and it assists your muscles as they repair themselves. Without a properly functioning immune system, you would be constantly sick and in bed instead of healthy and energetic. That's how significant the function of your immune system is.

Being aware of - and taking care of - this powerhouse defense system within your body is what ultimately makes you less susceptible to diseases. And although the immune system is a complex subject to discuss, this book is going to teach you (in a very easy-to-understand manner) exactly what you need to do to keep your immune system strong and operating optimally so that you can stay healthy and fit, enjoying a better quality of life.

Chapter 1: Understanding the Immune System and Innate Immunity

The immune system involves the lymphatic system and is composed of the thymus gland, spleen, lymph nodes, lymphocytes (B and T), lymphatic vessels and the lymph fluid. All these are involved in helping your body withstand "invasion" by disease-causing microbes and toxic chemicals. The major organ involved in the lymphatic system for immunity is the thymus gland.

What is the thymus gland?

It is a gland responsible for producing lymphocytes—the B and T. These are the cells responsible for protecting your body. The lymphocytes enter the bloodstream where they are activated for immune responses.

What is immunity?

This is the ability of the body to resist infectious microbes and toxic substances.

There are two types of immunity

1. Innate immunity

This immunity is characterized by a general response of the body to invading foreign materials (microbes and chemicals). This denotes that the body has the same response every time the infecting agent attacks.

2. Adaptive immunity

This is the type of immunity in which the body tends to improve its response each time the infecting agent attacks. In this type of immunity, the body responds more quickly because it remembers the infecting agent.

Factors involved in innate immunity

Chemical mediators

These are substances found on the surface of cells that are responsible for killing microbes or engulfing toxic chemicals. Examples are lysozymes that are found in saliva, tears and the mucus membranes of the nose. When you feel down, it's actually good to cry so you can

6

eliminate those harmful bacteria from your eyes. There are also interferons, which protect you from viruses. Other examples are leukotrienes that promote phagocytosis.

Phagocytosis is a process that involves the engulfment of foreign substances and harmful chemicals by the body cells.

Mechanical mechanisms

These mechanisms involve the skin and mucus membranes. They prevent infecting organisms and chemicals from entering the body. You can just imagine how easily a bacterium can enter your internal organs if it weren't for your skin covering. Bacteria would feast on all your vital organs and infect you easily.

Your urine, saliva, sweat and tears are parts of your immune system too because they act as your first line of defense. Urine helps eliminate toxic waste products of metabolism, while your saliva, sweat and tears wash away any microbes inhabiting the area.

Complements

These are substances that are protein in nature. They help in the phagocytosis and lysis (destruction) of bacterial cells to kill them.

White Blood Cells (WBC)

The WBCs are the most important cells in your immune system. They are produced in the bone marrow and the lymphatic system and they circulate through the blood. When the WBCs detect foreign substances they move towards them and isolate them through the process called chemotaxis.

Types of WBCs that help in the immune response of the body

- **Neutrophils**—These cells are like 911 cells because they arrive at the scene of infection first. They phagocytize the invading material quickly and prevent further infection. They respond quickly but they also die promptly after engulfing a foreign substance or bacteria.

- **Basophils and eosinophils**—These cells are responsible for causing inflammation so that infecting agents are killed. The substances released by these cells that cause inflammation must be controlled by other body mechanisms. This is to prevent the spread of the inflammation and to contain it within the boundaries of the destructive agent's influence. This also prevents the contamination of the other body parts.

- **Macrophages**—These are the cells that respond after neutrophils. They usually leave the bloodstream and go to the site of infection to phagocytize microbes and chemicals harmful to the body. They are typically found in major areas where infecting agents may enter, such as the skin.

Chapter 2: What Is Adaptive Immunity?

Adaptive immunity is formed when the body remembers and reacts specifically to a microorganism or to chemicals/substances it has previously encountered. The good thing about adaptive immunity is its ability not only to remember, but also improve on its immune response to infective agents. Adaptive immunity works though the following:

Antigens

These are substances that react with antibodies to help in the function of the immune system. It can be classified as self-antigens or foreign antigens. Self-antigens are formed inside the body while the foreign antigens are those coming from microorganisms or foreign substances invading the body.

There are two types of antigen response through the adaptive immunity

1. **Cell mediated immunity**

   Lymphocytes, specifically the B and T lymphocytes, act as defense systems through phagocytosis. In this response, the body develops immunity through the blood cells.

A special lymphocyte called the Natural Killer (NK) cells work by releasing chemicals that can destroy or lyse the membranes of the infecting agent. But, it does not remember previous exposures, so it reacts the same way no matter how many times the body has been exposed to the same agent.

2. Humoral immunity

The body develops immunity through the humors (body fluids). Body fluids include saliva, tears, sweat, urine, blood, vaginal and urethral secretions.

Antibodies

The body develops immunity when invading microorganisms (bacteria, fungi or viruses) cause the body to form antibodies in response to the microorganisms' antigen. Antibodies typically deactivate the antigen of the foreign substance to make it incapable of multiplying. This action can contain the spread of infection and cause the death of the invading organism.

Antibodies are specific. They only react with their specific antigens. So, there is no antibody that can go against all diseases. Each disease's antigen produces its own antibodies. When a person is exposed to that disease, he can develop the antibodies in his system. Next time the disease attacks again, the body will have antibodies that can defend it from the disease.

Helper T cells

These cells help both the cell-mediated and humoral systems to function effectively. It acts as the potential bridge that connects both systems so they can work together as one in ensuring that your body is protected from simple infections.

The above information about adaptive immunity has been the basis used by scientists in developing vaccines that produce antibodies inside your body to inactivate the infecting agent. Originally, vaccines were actual live organisms that have been weakened. Nowadays, the immunization products are safer because of alternative means of producing the antigens.

Chapter 3: What Is Acquired Immunity?

Acquired immunity is a type of adaptive immunity, which you develop after being exposed to a certain microorganism or chemical. It can be classified into:

1. **Natural**

   This is the type of immunity that you can acquire naturally through the contraction of the disease. It can be further classified into:

   Active natural—You develop immunity through your natural exposure to the infecting agent. This immunity develops after the person is personally exposed to the disease.

   Passive natural—This is when antibodies from a pregnant or lactating mother are transferred to the fetus or baby. The newborn baby relies on the mother's antibodies during the first few months of his life. After 6 months, the mother's antibodies are gone and the baby has to rely on his own antibodies.

2. Artificial

Active artificial—In this type of immunity, antigens are introduced deliberately through vaccines. Vaccines are composed of the infective microorganisms in their weakened forms. Their introduction to the body produces antibodies that will remain in your body. During a second infection, these antibodies will then be able to deactivate the invading microorganism's antigens and weaken the symptoms of the disease.

Passive artificial—In this type of immunity, antigens produced by an animal or another person are injected into you to produce antigens to that disease.

These are the ways your body develops immunity from the outside. In certain cases, vaccination may be the best choice, especially for babies and young children.

Chapter 4: When Your Immune System Is Impaired

When your immune system is impaired, your body's defenses are down, so infections can occur easily. You will be susceptible to all diseases you find yourself exposed to. There are diseases that can damage your immune response such as, Acquired Immune Deficiency Syndrome (AIDS) or Human Immunodeficiency Virus (HIV). In this condition, the virus damages your immune system by destroying your blood cells.

The following occurs when your immune system is impaired

1. **Susceptibility to diseases**

   When your immune system is down—as with AIDS/HIV—your body's defenses are weak. There's no barrier to stop the infecting agents from entering your body. Simply put, your body is like a palace without its royal guards (defense system). Anyone can enter and kill the king and queen (organs). This is the reason why AIDS/HIV patients are isolated because they can contract any disease that they come in contact with.

Getting sick easily is a symptom that your immune system is down. If you have intermittent bouts of sickness, consult your doctor immediately to determine the root cause. Your health must take the forefront in this case.

2. Poor wound healing

When your immune system is down, you don't have internal 911 responders, so your wounds won't heal as they normally do. You can bleed to death even with small cuts because there will be no white blood cells and platelets that can clot the wound. Your skin is your first line of defense therefore, treat your injuries promptly. Poor wound healing can lead to more serious infections and complications.

3. Organ failure

With the onset of various illnesses, organ failure can occur. It will be a free-for-all arena for bacteria, fungi and viruses to attack your major organs until they are decimated to tiny, useless pieces of flesh.

4. Death

When organ failure occurs, and no therapy or medical relief is provided, death is inevitable. When a serious illness attacks you and you don't have antibodies to counter it, this, too, is fatal.

An impaired immune system is life-threatening. It is a condition that you must avoid. Instead, find ways to improve and boost your immune system. This is your only option if you want to stay healthy.

Chapter 5: How to Give Your Immune System a Boost

After learning the facts about your immune system, it is equally important to know how to maintain and promote its health. Keep in mind that anything that damages cells or tissues can damage the immune system. The steps below will help you boost your immune system.

Step #1—Acquire a positive way of thinking

Believe it or not, thinking positively in any given situation is one definite way to boost your immune system. This is due to the fact that when you think positively, your brain commands the body to respond accordingly. It's your brain that stimulates your hormones to respond. It produces physical manifestations in your body that can influence your immune system. The brain is a powerful tool that controls all your body's systems, so feed it only with positive thoughts and good "food".

A positive way of thinking reduces stress and prevents the increased secretion of the stress hormone glucocorticoids. How reduction of stress can boost your immune system is presented in step #2.

Step #2—Cope with stress effectively

This is connected to your being an optimist. You will most likely agree that when you think positively, you will feel less stressed, because you will worry less. Worrying less will prevent the secretion of hormones such as epinephrine and norepinephrine that can elevate your blood pressure and exert undue pressure on your organs and on your immune system.

Stress also increases the secretion of your glucocorticoids that can affect the thymus which produces your lymphocytes. Glucocorticoid is a stress hormone produced by the adrenal glands that plays a detrimental role in the immune system. It inhibits vital substances such as, interleukins and cytokines. These two substances are vital in the activity of white blood cells—the primary cells involved in your immune response.

Learn how to cope with stress and how to relax daily. There are numerous techniques you can employ to relax yourself. Yoga, meditation and breathing exercises are the most common options.

Set aside time every day just to sit and relax in order to free yourself of stress. Breathing in and out deeply for a few minutes can relax you. Doing some muscle stretches for a few minutes can also do the trick.

Step #3—Eat more fruits and vegetables

Your immune system thrives on the cells that can properly perform their functions. These cells rely on your diet to stay strong and healthy. Studies have established that fruits and vegetables are beneficial to a person's health. This is because they are rich in essential nutrients that the body needs, sufficient fiber for gut health, and vitamins needed for cells, tissues and organs' development and growth.

Fruits, especially citrus fruits, and vegetables such as mushrooms and green leafy vegetables can also provide vitamins A, B, C, D, and E that your immune system needs. They contain chlorophyll and anti-oxidants that help cells stay healthy. They can also provide the minerals that your body needs such as potassium, magnesium, chloride, sodium, calcium and phosphorus.

Step #4—Don't drink alcohol

Your immune system depends significantly on the proper function of your cells, which is damaged by alcohol. When these body cells are impaired, your immune system is damaged too. Acetaldehyde, one of the end products of alcohol metabolism, has been found to cause liver cirrhosis. This toxic substance slowly kills cells and renders them keratinized or dead.

It's like you're committing suicide slowly and deliberately.

Aside from that, alcohol is a central nerve depressant that can diminish the normal function of your body's systems. This can lead to dysfunctions in your whole body including your immune system. You wouldn't want to keep drinking alcohol if you value your body and your health.

Step #5—Exercise daily

You may have read this advice several times, and may even think it's overrated. The fact remains, that you can never run away from exercise if you want to boost your immune system. Exercise is one of the inevitable pillars of good health. When you exercise, your blood circulation improves and your cells are adequately nourished. Remember that your white blood cells are the major cells involved in your immune system, hence if they are properly nourished, they can function effectively. Also, when you exercise, you sweat a lot. Sweating is one action of the immune system to get rid of microbes and toxic substances from your body. Furthermore, exercise can prevent obesity and keep you at your ideal weight. Sweat it out and help your immune system clean up your body. Exercise those muscles daily and let the blood flow smoothly in your blood vessels throughout your body.

Walk, jog, cycle, do aerobics or engage in sports to exercise those muscles and strengthen your defenses. It doesn't matter what type of exercise you engage in as long as you flex those muscles and work up a sweat. This can take from 30 minutes to one hour daily.

Step #6—Get enough sleep

It's when you sleep that some important substances and hormones are released sufficiently. Examples of these are Growth Hormone (GH) and Growth Hormone Releasing Hormone (GHRH). These hormones are important aspects in the growth of your cells and tissues. Anything that impedes the growth of cells will always impede the development of your immune system too.

Outside of your immune system, lack of sleep has many detrimental effects that can be fatal. Your brain is impaired too, affecting the normal functions of your body systems. Children need 8 to 10 hours sleep, while adults need at least 7 to 8 hours of sleep.

Step #7—Avoid bad fats, excess sugar and excess salt

Bad fats come from meat fat and dairy products, while good fats come from fruits and vegetables. Fats can cause various diseases such as, cardiac and liver disease. Bad fats can also weaken your immune system.

Too much sugar and salt can also damage your cells and tissues, and thereby, your immune system. Sugar in blood comes from carbohydrates such as, rice, pasta and bread, so don't overeat and make yourself sick. Salt comes from your plain table salt and is typically present in high levels in processed food. Taking too much salt can weaken your immune system because the water-electrolyte balance will not be maintained.

Step #8—Avoid illicit drugs

Drugs of abuse attack the cells of your body and destroy them. Take note that your major immunity players are your WBC, lymphocytes, neutrophils and eosinophils, which are all blood cells. Therefore, if these are all attacked by the components of your illicit drugs, then your immune system will be weakened significantly. Illicit drugs can affect your brain too and can harm your central nervous system. Plus—you risk jail time by using these addictive drugs. So, stay away from them!

Step #9—Don't smoke or drink too much coffee

The nicotine in cigarettes is harmful to blood cells. In fact, it destroys your respiratory cells and can cause lung cancer and other lung diseases. It can do the same damage to the cells of your immune system.

In the same manner that nicotine is bad for you, coffee can only cause harm in the long term. The caffeine in coffee can wake you up because it stimulates your hormones, but too much of it can have unhealthy repercussions. Both nicotine and caffeine tend to be addictive so these substances must be avoided.

Step #10—Take probiotics

A healthy gut will boost your immune system, so consume probiotics that contain healthy bacteria for your stomach. These bacteria (lactobacilli) are part of the normal flora of your stomach. They drive out the pathogenic microbes. Taking probiotics will help maintain the balance of the good bacteria inside your gut, consequently resulting in a better performing immune system. Probiotics is typically found in yogurt and other special beverages.

Step #11—Add more protein in your diet

Your antibodies are protein in nature, so protein in your diet can help boost your immune system. In addition, the amino acids coming from your protein diet are the building blocks of the growth and development of your cells. Sans these amino acids, you can't grow a single cell in your body. Examples of proteins are lean meat, soya beans, fish and egg white.

Step #12—Maintain a healthy social life

Scientists have confirmed that being able to live a happy social life, and being able to develop meaningful relationships can boost your immune system. This stems from the fact that when you have a healthy social life you tend to be happier and less stressed. With these positive emotions, your immune system is given a boost because your cells are produced properly without any interruptions from stress and unhappiness.

So, when you ask the question: how can these feelings affect your immune system? Remember that all emotions are sent to your brain and the brain reacts to manage them by stimulating the glands to produce specific hormones.

Studies also established that T cell functions have increased in people who have had successful relationships. Likewise, the antibody, IgG, increases when people socialize more. IgG fights off infections together with the other immunoglobulins.

Chapter 6: Important Lifestyle and Dietary Changes

In addition to the tips from the preceding chapter, here are important guidelines that you can refer to at home to further improve your immune system.

1. **Include the following ingredients in your menu planning:**

   - Garlic—promotes activity of white blood cells. Eat it raw for a more potent effect.

   - Onion—breaks up mucus and increases blood circulation. Include generous amounts in salads uncooked for better effects.

   - Ginger—acts as an inflammatory substance and good for flu. You can turn it into hot tea to help ease sore throat.

   - Olive oil—helps in providing good fat to your body so that cells can grow properly.

- Pepper—promotes growth of white blood cells. It helps you sweat, helping in the function of your immune system.

- Ginseng—is commonly believed to enhance the immune system, although more conclusive studies will yet confirm this claim.

- Aloe vera—has been helpful in treating burns and minor wounds.

- Pure honey bee—has been used in helping the immune system treat colds, and sore throat.

These natural products are used locally to strengthen—not only the immune system—but the whole body as well. They have anti-microbial and healing properties, and can be safely ingested. They are also inexpensive. Be sure to check for allergies to stay safe.

2. Instruct family members to observe proper hygiene.

Common sense dictates that you have to be clean to avoid acquiring infection. Observe proper hygiene by taking a bath daily, brushing your teeth at least twice a day, and washing your hands before and after meals. It's universally established that washing the hands with soap and water frequently is the best way to prevent infection.

Create an awareness of this healthy habit within your family. Of course, you can always include other people in your noble intention. Your end-goal is to stay uninfected and well. When you maintain your health, you also help your immune system to develop properly. Staying healthy will improve your immune system in the long run.

On the other hand, don't be afraid to expose your children to the environment. Allow them to play outside amidst the grass, dirt or soil, so their bodies can develop some antibodies on their own. A clean countryside is a good place to do this, not in a slimy, dirty and polluted neighborhood.

Decide wisely. If there's potential danger of contracting pathological diseases, then refrain from exposing them. You would not leave your children playing in a clean stream, if you know that malaria abounds in that area. Likewise, you will not allow your them to play in a gutter that can be infected with H-fever mosquito vectors.

3. Get a regular dose of early morning sunshine

Expose yourself to early morning sunshine for a healthy dose of Vitamin D. These are the light rays that are gentle to your skin. You can do this when the sun is still starting to rise on the horizon and its rays are not hot. This can be around 6 to 7:30 am. Don't go beyond that because too much sun exposure can lead to skin cancer.

Early sunshine activates the precursor of your vitamin D so that it can be converted into an active form. This activated vitamin D promotes skin health, thereby, improving your immune system. Remember that your skin is one of the components of your immune system, being your first line of defense.

4. Take good care of your skin

It goes without saying that you have to take good care of your skin and ensure that it's clean. You can use light moisturizers to prevent dryness and irritation. Treat skin sores and wounds promptly so they do not get infected. If you have diabetes mellitus, work with your doctor to manage the condition and promote better wound healing.

5. Cry, if you must

Have you ever wondered why you feel better after crying? This is because tears cleanse the eyes in addition to releasing pent up emotions. Tears wash away microbes from your eyes so don't hold back your tears. Cry whenever you feel like it.

6. Make love regularly

Yes, Virginia, making love regularly can help improve your immune system. There's a scientific connection that researchers were able to establish. An immunoglobulin, particularly salivary IgA, was found to increase in production in people who made love more. The immunoglobulins, are antibodies, and therefore part of your immune system.

7. Nurture a pet

If you're alone at home, consider caring for a pet. Developing a bond with a pet can bring peace and relaxation for you. This will reduce your stress and help improve your immune system, as it does when you socialize.

8. Strengthen family bonds

Your immune system improves when you have strong family ties. It's because stress is greatly reduced within your home. When stress is reduced and managed, your immune system improves, as well. This has something to do with the stress hormones, glucocorticoids, and IgG.

These are home guides that you can implement to improve your immune system. Continue to build on this list with natural and safe activities that make you feel light and worry free as you progress on your journey to a stronger immune system.

Chapter 7: Other Useful Pointers

In this chapter, we look at some overlooked truths about caring for the immune system. Let these pointers guide you to make better food and lifestyle choices, and help you succeed in your endeavor to improve your immune system.

1. **Not all herbal products are what they claim to be.** If you're offered one, you have to ensure that this is FDA approved or has been cleared by a recognized health entity in your area. Make sure that you're not also allergic to any of its components.

2. **The natural way of boosting your immune system is still best**. There are enough natural techniques in this book that you can implement, so make use of them responsibly. Multivitamins can help you get there, but it's better to eat nutritious foods instead. If you can't eat fruits or vegetables because of a valid reason, you can resort to multivitamins but consult your doctor first.

3. **Very young and older individuals have weaker immune systems.** Pediatric and geriatric individuals are more prone to

sickness because their immune systems are not fully functioning. Pediatric persons are those less than 6 months old and geriatric persons are individuals who are more than 60 years old.

4. **Kiss judiciously**. Although you're encouraged to make love, you must ensure that you don't kiss persons you barely know. You have to observe personal hygiene even with your long time partners. Brushing your teeth before kissing may not always be feasible but is a good hygiene practice. Your saliva is where the microbes congregate to be washed away. Do not use your tongue to swipe away the millions of microbes from your partner's mouth.

5. **Undergo annual screening tests.** This will determine if your immune system's response is functioning reliably. Complete Blood Count, and peripheral blood smears can be performed to check if your counts are normal. The doctor will perform physical exam and may order other diagnostic exams, if necessary.

6. **Avoid drugs given to athletes to boost their immunity.** You may have heard of such

drugs. These are not officially approved by the health department. You must see the official stamp of the licensed certifying organization in your area before using them.

7. **Individuals with AIDS or HIV should seek medical treatment immediately.** If you have AIDS or HIV, you have to report to your health center ASAP. While there is still no cure for this disease, researchers have been able to develop a drug that can deter its growth. Your health center will help you in managing this condition.

8. **Prevention is always better than cure.** Get those vaccinations. You and your children should have complete vaccines such as, oral polio (OPV), diphtheria, pertussis, tetanus (DPT), and other safe vaccines. Tetanus can cause death in a non-vaccinated person. If you're unsure whether to give your child the vaccine, consult a competent pediatrician.

9. **Your immune system can fail at times.** It's not perfect. There are limits to what your immune system can do. There will be many times that your body gives in to an infecting microorganism. This is why, even if your immune system is functioning well, it is best

to avoid coming in contact with infectious agents.

10. **Those delicious desserts can impair your immune system.** Curb your desire for cakes, ice creams, chocolates because they can cause obesity and weight problems. They can also cause hyperglycemia (increased blood glucose levels) which can damage your immune system.

Conclusion

The information on the immune system as presented here is vital to understanding how to strengthen the defense system against sickness. We tried to present it in a straightforward and simple way so that you and your family members (even the younger ones) can refer to this book at any time.

Utilize the recommended methods in this book properly and you will definitely improve your immune system and your health in general. Health is wealth and you have to put in time and effort in order to reap the benefits of a healthy body. Nothing good will happen unless you act on the information you got from this book.

It's important to note that there are a few techniques that should be implemented carefully, because the opposite can happen if the step is not followed correctly. You're encouraged to go back and double check the information in the various chapters, should you have doubts.

Finally, I'd like to thank you for purchasing this book! If you found it helpful, I'd greatly appreciate it if you'd take a moment to leave a review on Amazon. Thank you!